Bibliografische Information der Deutschen Nationalbibliothek:

Die Deutsche Bibliothek verzeichnet diese Publikation in der Deutschen Nationalbibliografie; detaillierte bibliografische Daten sind im Internet über http://dnb.d-nb.de/ abrufbar.

Impressum:

Druck und Bindung: Books on Demand GmbH, Norderstedt Germany
ISBN: 978-3-668-07151-3

Dieses Buch bei GRIN:

http://www.grin.com/de/e-book/308605/image-processing-applied-to-melanoma-detection

Elyoenai Guerra-Segura, Carlos M. Travieso-González, Jesús B. Alonso-Hernández

Image Processing Applied to Melanoma Detection

Designing an Automatic System with High Sensitivity

GRIN Verlag

Applying Image Processing to Melanoma Evaluation

Designing an automatic system with high sensitivity

Guerra-Segura, Elyoenai
Travieso-González, Carlos M.
Alonso-Hernández, Jesús B.

Abstract

This book tries to show the basic steps a classification system should take into account when trying to solve a classification problem. This does not mean all systems have to follow this guide. It only gives the normal steps to study when developing a classification system. In particular, this work shows the steps followed when applying a classification system in order to classify melanocytic lesions as melanoma or moles.

As mentioned before, this guide is based on a well-known problem. The problem studied is the classification of melanocytic lesions as melanocytic nevus or melanoma cancer. This work has been developed with the collaboration of *Hospital Universitario de Gran Canaria Doctor Negrín*.

The idea of writing this guide is based on the results obtained and the systems applied. The main results has been published in [1]. In this guide all the particular process followed in order to get the published results is explained. The general steps of a classification system are only shown briefly.

Almost all the images are extracted from the original work and the paper named before. All the images shown in this guide were obtained by the authors.

All the original work was presented at *Universidad de Las Palmas de Gran Canaria* to obtain the degree of Telecommunications in 2014.

Table of contents

1. Introduction

1.1. Health and technology. E-Health.

Human being lives in a society which is continuously changing. This evolution can be observed in education, technology, health, etc. In this book we show an example of how health and technology evolution can change together looking for common goals. Both fields have started to work jointly to achieve a better quality of life. This cooperation has become so important that telemedicine is becoming a new concept called e-Health.

Telemedicine is a well-known concept which is mainly based on projects that use "Information and Communication Technologies (ICTs)" to connect doctors and patients in order to provide clinical health care at a distance. It also consists on a high data flow from different medical centers and professionals, which allows sharing knowledge and different case studies which could improve the global health status.

As an example of telemedicine, in late 1998 on the Canary island of *El Hierro* it was developed first pilot project undertaken by the *Servicio Canario de Salud.* The services of the Hospital de *La Candelaria* in Tenerife offered telecare within their disciplines telepsychiatry, teledermatology and teleradiology. Its rating obtained a higher level of satisfaction, 97% in the population served and a very high rating in the medical community who participated and made this experience possible.

However, e-Health is not only about telemedicine, but also covers all the new developments which have improved the quality of the diagnoses in hospitals. To achieve this, these developments usually use image and signal processing techniques [1].

1.2. Melanocytic diseases

Melanocytic diseases are produced by alterations of the melanocytes. Melanocytes are the cells which produces melanin (the primarily responsible for skin color). However, alterations of melanocytes could become malign or benign diseases.

Benign accumulations of melanocytes are known as melanocytic nevus, commonly called moles. They are the result of a controlled proliferation of the melanocytes. On the other hand, when the proliferation is uncontrolled, the results are malign diseases called melanomas.

Melanocytic diseases, as it has been shown, can be divided in the following two groups:

- Melanocytic nevus
- Melanomas

Melanocytic nevus can be also divided in subgroups attending to the moment the disease appears or to the characteristics. In this book we have worked with 6 kinds of melanocytic nevus, classified attending to their characteristics, which are presented in the chapter dedicated to the database.

Although Melanomas only represent the 4% of the skin tumors, they cause 80% of deaths [2, 3]. An early detection is very important. If the melanoma is removed when is lower than 1 mm, the patient will have a recovery in 90%-95% of cases [4,5].

To show the difficulty of melanoma diagnosis, in figure 1 a melanocytic nevus and a melanoma are shown, respectively.

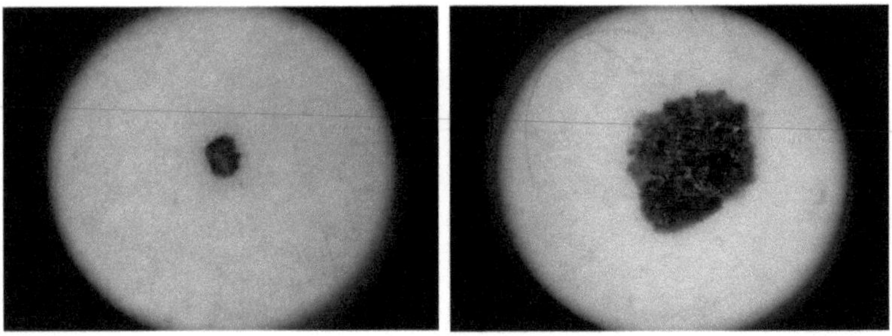

Figure 1. Melanocytic nevus and melanoma

1.3. Background

Once the problem is presented, we have to plan how to try solving it. First of all, take a look to both the previous works and the techniques they use.

The background could be divided into the following 3 groups, according to what stage of the image processing techniques they focus on:

Automatic lesion segmentation: these works have been developed in order to increase the efficiency of the automatic segmentation of the lesion. This in the one of the most important steps when applying automatic algorithms to solve problems like the one we are trying to solve. These algorithms try to detect the region of interest (ROI) in the image, since it will be the region to evaluate later. Two examples of this group are shown in [6–8].

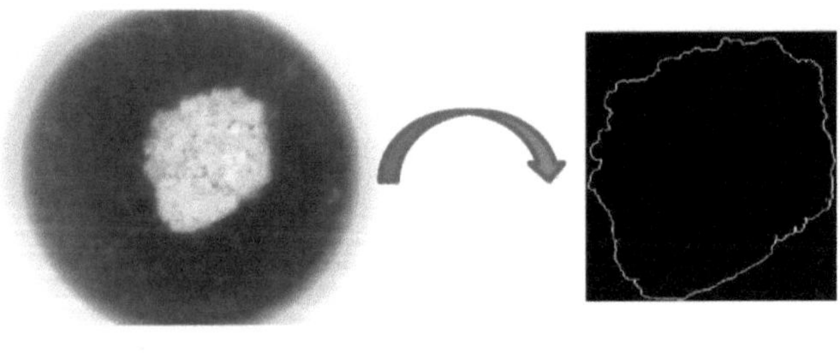

Figure 2. Border detection of a melanocytic disease

Evaluation of dermatologist characteristics: the second group is about the works which apply different dermatological rules. One of these rules is called ABCD rule and it is a well-known technique and one of the most used by the dermatologist. Seven-point checklist is another dermatological rule which is also usually implemented by these techniques. These rules try to evaluate difference characteristics of the lesion, as dermatologists do. Some examples of these works are shown in [9,10].

Automatic classifier based on feature extraction techniques: this third group is composed of works which are based on the use of automatic classifiers. As it is shown in figure 3, the basic schematic of these works are based on the feature extraction step. These works start from the ROI obtained with the segmentation step and extract the features from it. Once the features are extracted, they are used in a classifier for training and testing. In a future chapter this schematic and each of its steps will be explained. Some examples of these works are shown in [1,10–18].

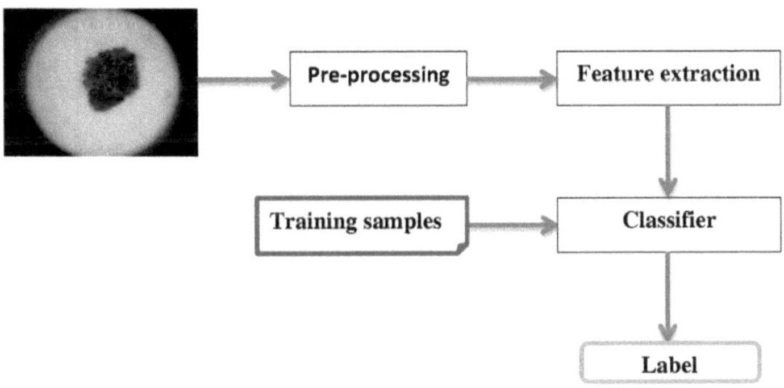

Figure 3. Schematic of a typical automatic classifier system

If we look at the 3 groups, some questions are logical:

- What features are extracted in the feature extraction step?
- Is it always necessary to segment the lesion to extract these features?

The work we are going to develop is going to use parts from the 3 groups as it is indicated below:

1. Image segmentation based on the best algorithms from group number 1.
2. Characteristics evaluated in group number 2 in order to develop the algorithms for the feature extraction.
3. Automatic classifier as in group number 3, using the features extracted.

1.4. Structure of the chapters

Based on the 3 groups shown above, the system has to implement an image segmentation step. Once we have the ROI in the image, we have to extract its characteristics based on the characteristics evaluated by the dermatologists, as group number 2 does. Finally, we have to use the features extracted to run an automatic classifier in order to label an input image as melanoma or melanocytic nevus.

To explain how to do this, step by step, the book is divided in the following chapters:

1. **Introduction**: brief introduction to the problem and the background.
2. **Theoretical foundations**: introduction to the dermoscopies, the dermatoscope and the ABDC rule.
3. **Database and image processing**: characteristics of the lesions, the images and the basic knowledge about image processing to be able to develop the system. The image pre-processing and segmentation steps are explained here.
4. **Feature extraction**: characteristics extracted from the images. The characteristics to extract based on ABCD rule and how to draft the algorithms.
5. **Classifier**: brief chapter about the used classifier and some bibliography for the readers.
6. **Feature selection**: explanation of how to select the characteristics which give more discriminant information about the lesions.
7. **Results**: obtained results from the different simulations and how to interpret them. It is also shown how to increase the results according with the needs of the system.

2. Theoretical foundations

In this chapter, the basic theoretical foundations needed to understand the importance of dermoscopies and the tool used to capture them are explained. The base of ABCD rule is also shown. Moreover, the characteristics evaluated by the doctors and the limitations of developing an automatic system based on it are explained too. The features extracted by the previous works are detailed and a draft of the system to develop is finally planed.

2.1. Dermatoscope and dermoscopy

The diagnosis of a melanocytic disease depends on the human eye and the optical properties of the skin. Sometimes, trying to give a diagnosis using the clinical eye could become a tedious work. However, there are some techniques which help doctors to get a better image of the lesion. One of those techniques is called dermoscopy.

Dermoscopies are the examination of the skin with a dermatoscope. This technique combines a method which makes the cornea layer translucent with an optical help increasing the projected image of the lesion on the retina. In figure 4 we can observe an image of a melanocytic lesion and a dermoscopy of the same lesion.

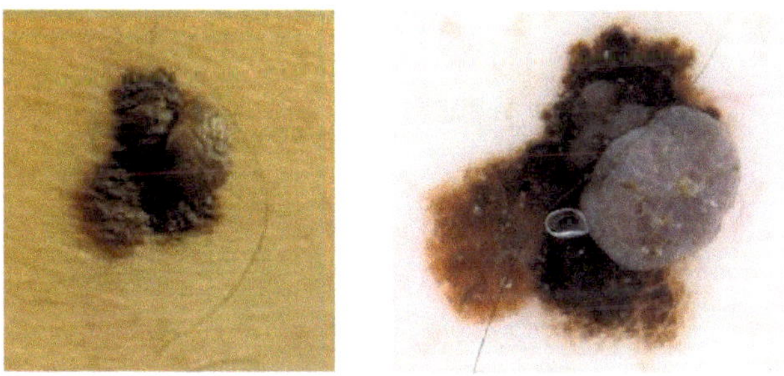

Figure 4. Clinical image and dermoscopy

It is a complementary technique to the clinical exploration. It is a noninvasive technique, economic and easy to implement with the appropriated tools. The use of the dermatoscope is being increase in different medical fields due to the possibility to observe characteristics which are not visible for the human eye.

2.1.1. The technique

One of the main problems when observing a melanocytic lesion is the reflection in the interface air-cornea layer. This effect limits the vision of the tissues located under the surface and gives little information about the possible structures presented on the lesion.

The objective of this technique is to avoid the effects of the reflection and the refraction produced when the light falls on the lesion. To make it possible, it can use cross polarized light or non-polarized light to use liquid immersion dermoscopies.

Dermoscopy combines a method which makes the cornea layer translucent with an optical help to improve the vision. This technique increases the observable morphological details.

The dermatoscope used in the *Servicio de Dermatología del Hospital Universitario de Gran Canaria Doctor Negrín* was the **DermLite II hybrid** m.

2.2. ABCD rule

This rule was developed by Stolz and other researchers at the University of Regensburg (Germany) in 1994. It is based on a multivariable analysis of four dermatological characteristics and it is a simple method.

This rule should be used when it has been diagnoses that the lesion is melanocytic.

Standard ABCD dermatologic protocol has been source of numerous features extraction algorithms. According to each of the four evaluated aspects through the rule (Asymmetry, Borders, Color and Dermoscopic structures), the TDS (Total Dermoscopy Score) is calculated. To get the TDS value, the formula is obtained as follows:

$$\mathbf{TDS = A \times 1.3 + B \times 0.1 + C \times 0.5 + D \times 0.5} \quad (1)$$

2.2.1. Features of ABCD

As mentioned above, the four features evaluated with this rule are:

Assymetry

To evaluate this features, lesions are divided in two axis of 90° collocated to obtain the minimum score of asymmetry. This feature is evaluated according to color, shape and structures present in both sides. The score goes from 0 to 2 depending on how many asymmetry axes the lesion has. In figure 5, possible axes are shown.

3 pairs of asymmetry are shown, what makes a total number of 6 axes. The normal axes are vertical and horizontal as the first pair. The second pair usually is formed of the main diagonal and its perpendicular. And the third pair consists of the second diagonal and its perpendicular. Note that dermoscopies rarely are square images. The evaluation should be done once the lesion is oriented respect to the horizontal.

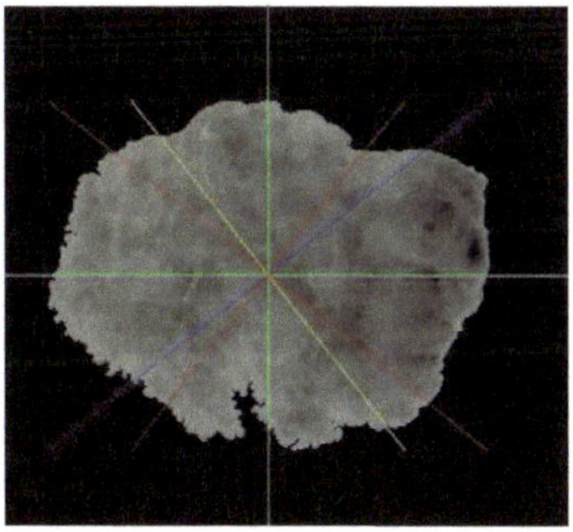

Figure 5. Example of possible axes to evaluate the asymmetry

Borders

In this feature, the abruptness of the borders is evaluated. The lesion usually is divided in 8 segments, what makes the score goes from 0 to 8. Benign lesions tend to finish abruptly.

Color

This characteristic evaluates the number of colors presented on the lesion. Many colors presented mean less symmetry in the growth of the cells, so the lesions could be malignant. Evaluated colors usually are black, white, gray-blue, red, dark brown, light brown. The score goes from 1 to 6.

Dermatoscopic structures

This feature evaluates the presence of 5 dermatoscopic structures. The score goes from 0 to 5.

Once the 4 scores are calculate, they are multiplied by the corresponding correction factors according with the equation 1.

Lesions are classified in 3 groups according to the TDS obtained, as shown in table 1:

TDS	Group
TDS < 4.75	Benign
4.75< TDS < 5.45	Suspicious
5.45 > TDS	Malignant

Table 1. Classification according to the TDS

2.2.2. Problems of the rule

The evaluation of the rule seems to be simple. However, how could we automatize it?

First of all, image segmentation techniques have to be applied to detect the ROI to evaluate. Later, image processing techniques should be applied in order to evaluate the four features of the rule.

But, when trying to quantify the lesion according to ABCD rule and its 4 characteristics, there are some problems difficult to solve. Some of these problems are listed below:

What is the threshold to label an axis as asymmetric? Once the axes are collocated and the two halves of the image are compared according to their colors, shapes, structures, what quantity of similitude is needed to label that axis as symmetric or asymmetric?

About borders, for each of the 8 segments we have to decide if its termination is abruptness or it is not. Moreover, the evolution of the radius along the border should be also computed. So, for each of the 8 segments we have to set a threshold to unify the abruptness and the evolution of the radius to label each segment as 1 or 0.

Color feature presents similar problems. On the on one hand, what percentage of pixels means a color is present on the lesion? On the other hand, how to label all possible colors to one of the 6 colors evaluated with this rule?

Finally, dermatoscopic structures follow a very subjective evaluation. It depends on the experience of the doctors and automatic evaluations of the presence of different structures have been a problem for years. The evaluation of the features usually is substituted by the evaluation of the diameter. However, when using dermoscopies it is not possible this evaluation since we do not know the distance or the focus.

We can observe there are several problems to solve in order to apply the ABCD rule in the same way dermatologist do. They are able to do this due to their clinical experience.

Although it is difficult to apply ACBD rule according to TDS formula, it is possible to develop an automatic classification system based on the same features ABCD rules evaluates. It means that the feature extraction step of a normal automatic classification system could be developed in order to extract characteristics about the asymmetry, the borders, the color and the presence of dermatoscopic structures.

In the next point, the most used features in the background are shown.

2.3. Features used in the background

As we have seen before, ABCD rule is indicates what features are usually evaluated when diagnosing melanocytic lesions. However, its automatic development presents several problems very difficult to solve.

If we look to the background of this filed, different works have applied automatic classification systems based on ACBD rule. Some of these works are shown in [1,9-11,13-17]

To detail the features, we can group them in 5 main groups, as it is shown below:

Symmetry

Several works focus on features related with this characteristic of the ABCD rule [9, 11-12]. This is because it shows an uncontrolled growth of cells which can lead to melanoma cancer. In [12], a study of the optimal axes to evaluate the symmetry is shown. Some of the proposed features to characterize this aspect are the *Asymmetry Index (AI)* and the *Lengthening Index (LI)*, computed to evaluate the overlapping area of both halves and the elongation of the lesion.

Border

Different proposals [4,13–15] try to evaluate the border characteristic of the rule using some methods like applying the gradient and the Laplacian to the borders, and then to characterize the results by the its averages, maximum and minimum values, etc. Using some numeric features as the *Irregularity Index*, this computes the area and the perimeter of the lesion. Borders could be also evaluated by computing the evolution of the radius along the lesion, looking for abruptness changes in the radius.

Color

This is the feature evaluated in almost all the works studied for the background. The main difference between the ways to compute it is based on the color channels used by the different works [9,16-17].

The goal of this feature is to evaluate the distribution of the channels. Some of these channels are Red-Green-Blue (RGB), Hue-Saturation-Value (HSV), Hue-Saturation-Intensity (HIS), and CIE Lab, which was defined by the *Commission Internationale de l'éclairage.*

Other difference presented in the different works is to evaluate the color of the lesion or to evaluate the color of the lesions and the color of the skin near the lesion.

It can also be evaluated according to different features like Compactness Index, Fractal Dimension, Edge Abruptness and Pigmentation Transition.

Dermatoscopic Structures

Most of the studied background refers to the difficulty to evaluate this aspect and propose different methods like to substitute it. One of these methods is to evaluate the texture of the lesion.

Texture

The texture offers information about the dermatoscopic structures presented in the lesions. Because of this, it is very used to substitute the D parameter of the ACBD rule [16,19]

It could be computed by applying the gradient to the lesion or different mathematics transformation to the image.

Diameter

Other way to substitute de D parameter is to compute the diameter of the lesion [4,9]. This way is not possible to apply in our case because the lack of information about the way the dermatoscopies were obtained, which mean there is no information about the scale and the diameter cannot be computed.

2.4. Proposed method for the diagnosis

Once we have presented the studied background and the main features related to ABCD rule, in this section we show the method to develop in order to diagnose dermatoscopic lesions.

The method follows the structure of an automatic classification system, based on features related to ABCD rule and using Support Vector Machine (SVM) as classifier.

The initial idea can be compressed into the flowchart shown below:

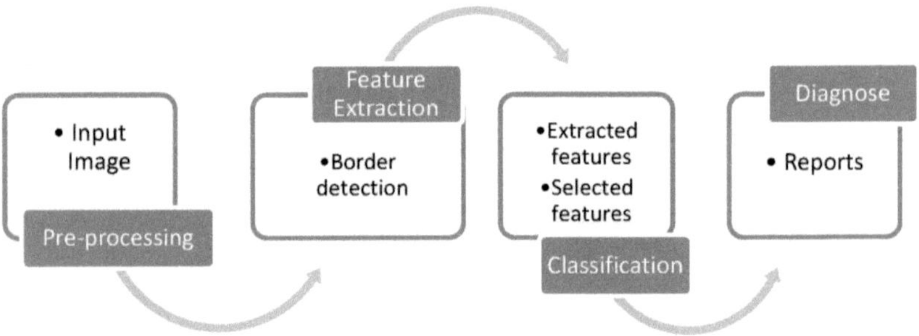

When applying the classification step it is necessary a previous database where the features of the different kind of lesions are stored in order to compare the new images with them. These features are the best ones to discriminate between benign and malignant lesions. The database is shown in chapter 3 and the features obtained are shown in chapter 4, while the best features are selected in chapter 6.

3. Database and image processing basis

In this chapter the used database is presented with its main characteristics.

Later an introduction to image processing and its typical steps is shown to get the basis to develop our system. From all the typical steps, we will focus on the feature extraction step.

3.1. Database

The final database used to develop this work contains 48 images, 24 of these images of benign lesions (of different kinds of nevus) and the other 24 images of malign lesions (melanomas and a kind of nevus which is usually label as malign).

The original database was generated by Dr. Carretero, *Head of Servicio de Dermatología* at *Hospital Universitario de Gran Canaria Doctor Negrín* and his team, with images from 124 patients.

We can observe that the original database was larger than the one used (at least it contains 124 images). The reason of this size reduction is that some of the images had poor quality and they had to be discarded.

The original database contained samples of the following kinds of lesions:

- Melanoma
- Compound Nevus
- Dysplastic Nevus
- Intradermal Nevus
- Junctional Nevus
- Reed Nevus
- Spitz Nevus

The original database was formed of 7 folders (one per each kind of lesion) with different numbers of patients. It was formed of clinical pictures and dermoscopies. In the table 2, the distribution of patients can be observed.

Kind of lesion	Number of patients
Melanoma	44
Compound Nevus	18
Dysplastic Nevus	13
Intradermal Nevus	18
Junctional Nevus	6
Reed Nevus	12
Spitz Nevus	13

Table 2. Patients distribution

From the total number of images we selected the dermoscopies where the lesion appears at all and correctly focused. Finally we obtained the 48 images of the final database, which have a distribution according to the kind of lesion as shown in table 3. There are no many dermoscopies since this kind of images are beginning to be obtained.

As it can be observed in table 3, both melanoma and dysplastic nevus are labeled as malign. Looking at the table we can observe the lesions and divided into 2 groups (benign and malign). There are 24 samples for each of the 2 groups, as mentioned above.

Kind of lesion	Number of samples	Diagnosis	Example
Melanoma	16	Malign	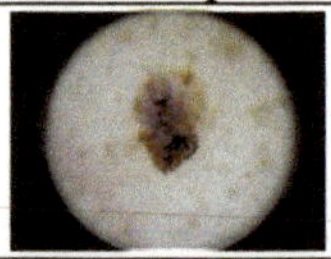
Compound Nevus	11	Benign	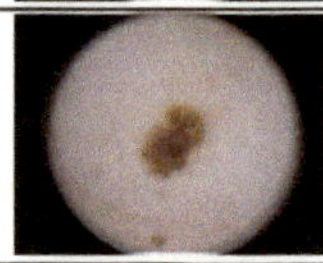
Dysplastic Nevus	8	Malign	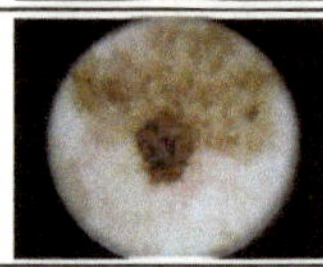
Intradermal Nevus	2	Benign	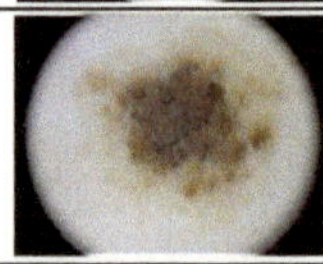
Junctional Nevus	4	Benign	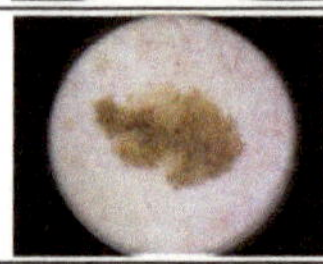
Reed Nevus	2	Benign	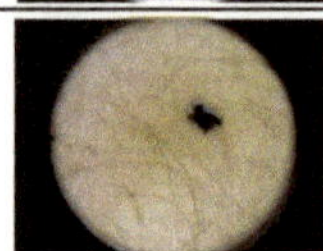
Spitz Nevus	5	Benign	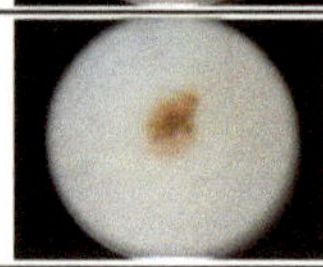

Table 3. Composition of the database

In table 4 we can resume the characteristics of the final database.

Parameters	Details from the final database
Number of classes	2
Number of samples per class	24
Acquisition and quantification	sRGB (24 bits, 256 leves per channel)
Size	2560 x 1920 pixels
Example	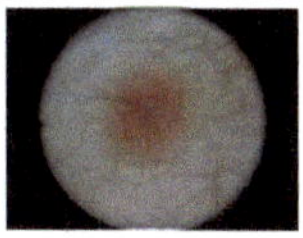

Table 4. Characteristics of the database

3.2. Introduction to image processing

Color digital images are formed of pixels, and the pixels are formed by combination of primary colors. A channel, in this context, is the image in grayscale and with the same size than the color image, made from one of these primary colors. For example, a picture taken with a normal digital camera has the red, green and blue channels (RGB channels), as shown in figure 6. A grayscale image has only one channel.

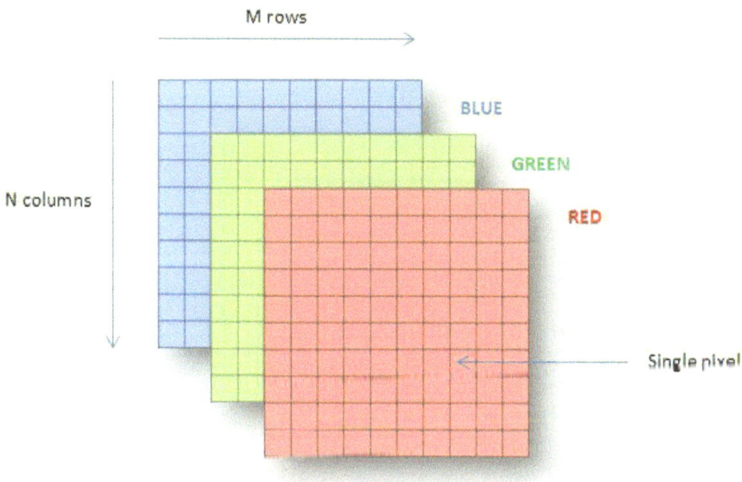

Figure 6. Matrix representation of RGB channels

In figure 6 we can observe how a RGB color image is consists of 3 matrixes of M rows and N columns. Each of these 3 matrixes represents one of the three RGB channels. At the same time, each of the matrixes is formed by pixels which can take different values depending of the intensity of the primary color. Finally, each of the pixels of the color images consists of 3 pixels which belong to the three RGB channels.

In figure 7 the separation of a color image into its 3 RGB channels is shown.

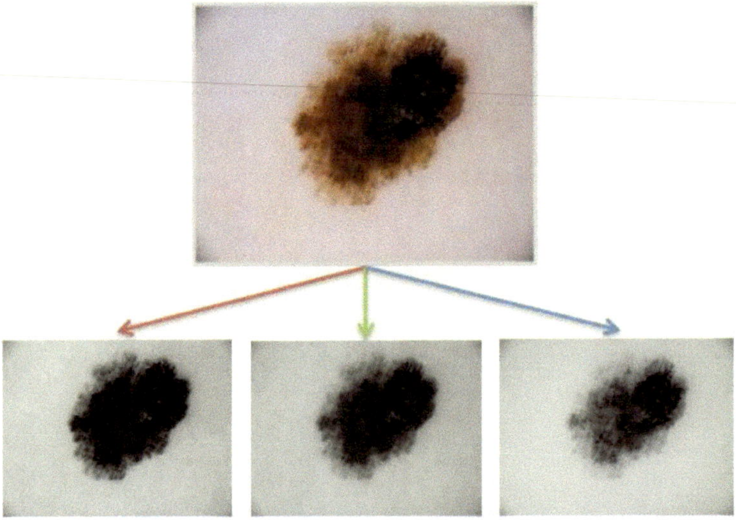

Figure 7. RGB separation of a dermoscopy image

As we show before, the image of the database were sRGB images with 24 bits. This means there 8 bits for each of the 3 channels. Each color image is composed of 3 grayscale images. One of this grayscale images has pixels which represent the intensity from 0 to 255.

Image processing is the group of techniques applied to digital images to improve the quality or make easier the information search. It high progress is also due to the advance of mathematics, computer science, the better knowledge of the organs which take part in image perception and manipulation, etc. The progress of image processing is reflected in medicine, geology, biology, astronomy, etc.

In figure 8 we can observe the typical steps of image processing.

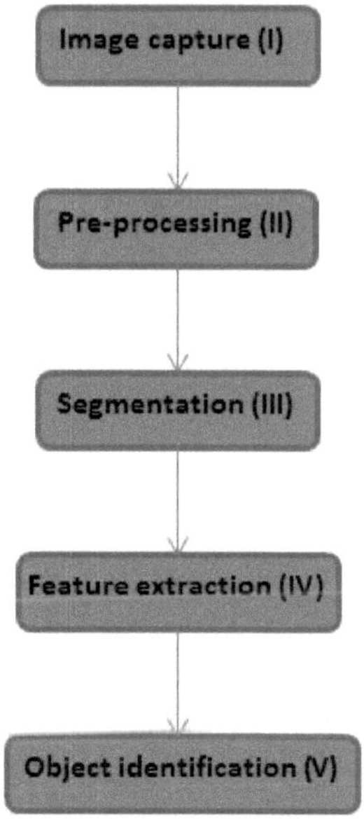

Figure 8. Typical steps of image processing

3.3. Image processing steps

As we work with digital images (dermoscopies), it is not necessary the image capture step. However, to try to avoid problems in the capture of the images, as the ones we observed (images were not focus, lesions does not appear entirely in the images, etc.) an image acquisition protocol is proposed here.

In this chapter we explain steps II and III while steps IV and V are shown in next chapters due its importance and particularities.

As we can observe in figure 8, pre-processing step is very important in order to have an acceptable segmentation. Its goals can be resumed as trying to adjust the quality of the image and highlighting the regions of interest as much as possible in order to develop a good segmentation step.

Segmentation step's importance is based on the fact we should identify correctly the region of interest of the image in order to obtain its features. In this case, we have to identify the lesions over the background to characterize it and extract the information to differentiate between the two classes we work with.

This information is extracted by applying the feature extraction step. This information is used in the last step of the process.

The last step in not an image processing step, this step processes the extracted features with the goal of identifying the image with one of the classes we have defined. In other words, this last step uses a classifier which relates the input image with the defined classes in order to obtain the similarities between them. In figure 9 we can observe a normal scheme of a classifier. As we can see, system (a) defines the classes from the labeled images. System (b) compares an input image with the known classes and gives a label according with the similarity between them. The classifier is explained in chapter 5.

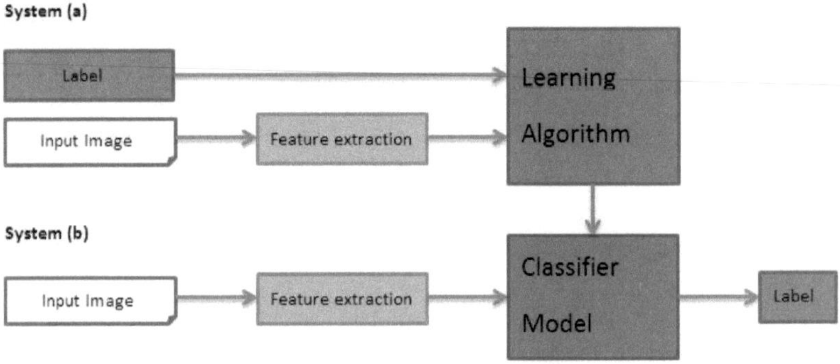

Figure 9. Classifier system scheme

3.4. Pre-processing and segmentation

In this section the pre-processing and segmentation steps are applied to the problem we are studying. We apply both steps as one since the main goal is adjust the quality of the image and detect the lesion over the background.

We can divide the section into 3 phases. The first one is noise removal. The second one is lesion detection, and the last phase is the contour extraction.

Before the 3 phases, the first step is to obtain the grayscales images from the input color image. This step is necessary since the morphological algorithms we are going to use works over two dimensional matrixes. So first of all we should apply *rgb2gray* Matlab function and normalize the new matrix so all possible grayscales images are in the same scale.

3.4.1. Noise removal

When working with dermoscopies, noise is mainly represented by hair over the area of the lesion which could disturb when extracting the contour of the lesion [20,21]. To remove possible hairs, we can use algorithms based on morphological operators as dilation and erosion [22]. Below, we show a basic algorithm which uses these two morphological operators and is able to get very good results depending on the structural element used (see figure 10). This algorithm is shown in order to readers can develop their own algorithms based on the characteristics of the images they use.

```
%structural element definition
se1 = strel('disk', 3);
%dilatation
BWe=imdilate(Im, se1);
BWe=imdilate(BWe, se1);
BWe=imdilate(BWe, se1);
%erosion
BWd=imerode(BWe, se1);
BWd=imerode(BWd, se1);
BWd=imerode(BWd, se1);
```

In the case of figure 10, 'Disk' has been chosen as the structural element.

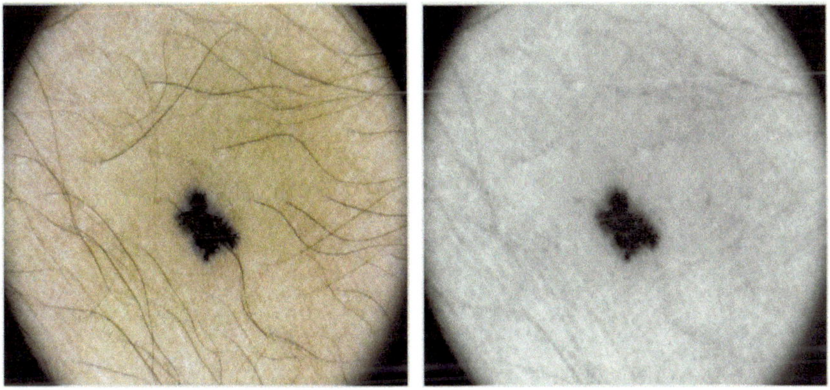

Figure 10. Result of hair removal algorithm. Input image to process and grayscale image after hair removal

Changing the kind of structural element and its size, different results are obtained according to the characteristics of the images. Size should be adjusted depending of the resolution of the images for example.

3.4.2. Lesion detection

Once grayscale image is normalized and possible hairs have been removed, an algorithm to detect the lesion has to be applied. To do this, we have to study the characteristics of the lesions we want to detect in order to develop an optimized algorithm for the problem.

All the dermoscopies of the database consist on dark centered lesions over light background. So the main goal of the lesion detection phase is to select the dark object of the middle of the image to process it later.

The easiest way is to binarizing the grayscale image and then, selecting the object with the nearest centroid to the middle of the image [23–25].

To binarizing the grayscale image there are a lot of different techniques which can be applied. The simplest way to use image binarization is to choose a threshold value, and classify all pixels with values above this threshold as white, and the rest as black. This is knows as technique based on threshold. How to select the best threshold is the question to solve.

One of the most used based on threshold techniques due to its good results is Otsu's method. This method chooses the optimal threshold by maximizing the between-class variance. It defines the between-class variance of the binarized image as [26]:

$$\sigma_B^2 = w_1(\mu_1 - \mu_T)^2 + w_2(\mu_2 - \mu_T) \quad (2)$$

where w_1 and w_2 are the probabilities of class occurrence, μ_1 and μ_2 are the mean intensities for classes 1 and 2 and μ_T is the mean intensity for the whole image.

However, if we look at the grayscale image shown in figure 10, we realize that when binarizing the image the lesions is becoming a black object over white background. This fact could be a problem depending on the functions we use to detect the objects and compute its centroids. To make this step easier, it is advisable to obtain the complementary image of the grayscale image and binarizing the new one to have white object over a black background, as shown in figure 11. To obtain the complementary image of a grasycale image, the *imcomplement* function can be used in Matlab.

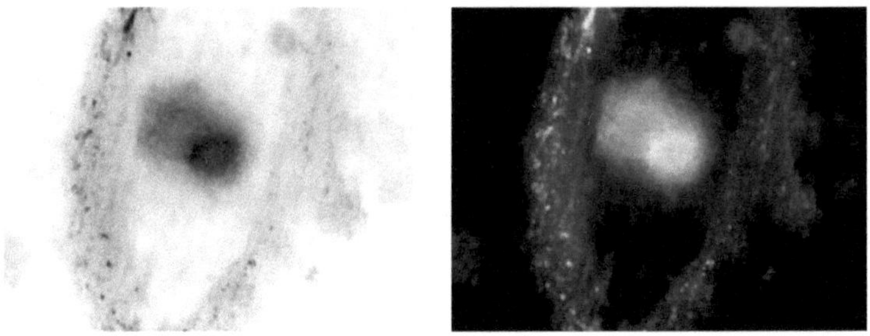

Figure 11. Grayscale image after noise removal and complementary image of the grayscale image

In figure 12, the histogram of image shown in figure 11 can be observed to understand the objective of the binarization algorithm. As we can observe, most of the pixels are near to 0. Looking at the image, we can guess all those pixels belong to the background.

In this example, if we apply Otsu's method using Matlab, the threshold y set at 78, very near no the dark grays area. Calculating the binarized image according to this threshold, the image shown in figure 13 is obtained.

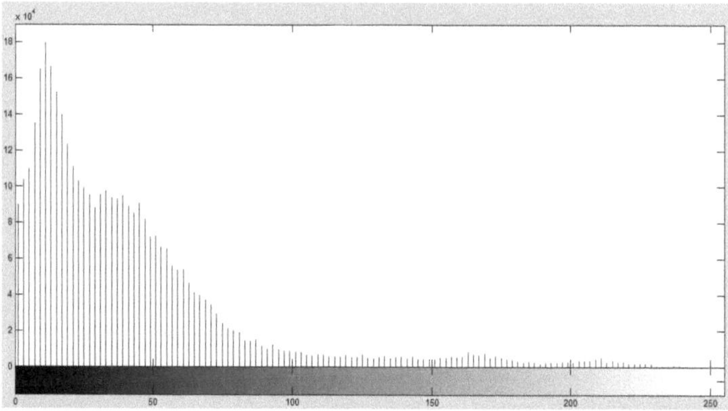

Figure 12. Histogram of the grayscale image shown in figure 11. The threshold is set at 78 by Otsu's method

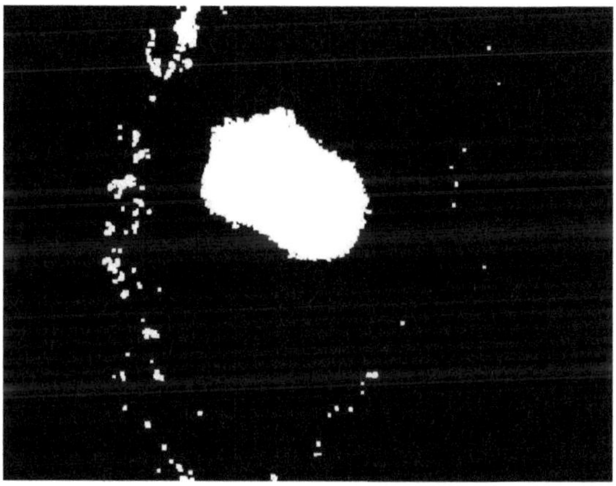

Figure 13. Binarized image obtained from image shown in figure 11 by applying Otsu's method

We can observe that the image in figure 13 shows a main big object in the middle. This is supposed to be the location and the characteristics of the lesion. In figure 14 the original image is shown in order to check that the lesion detection phase works accordingly with the characteristics of the images we are working with.

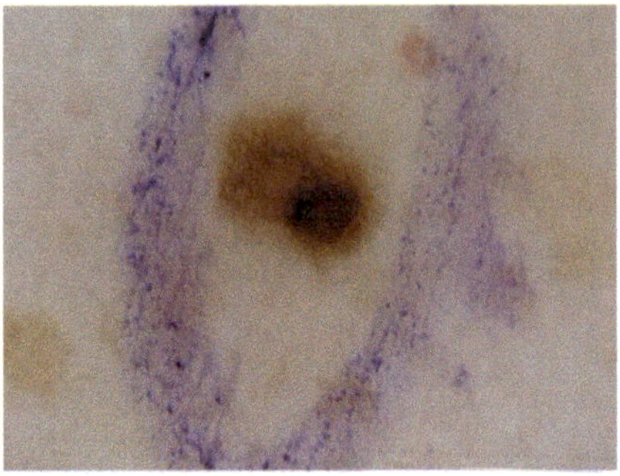

Figure 14. Original image processed to obtain the image of figure 13

It is shown the correctly performance of the binarization algorithm with the image of the example. However, there are some images which generate errors due to the black background around the original dermoscopy. One example of these cases is shown in figure 15. The problem is because black background, which does not belong to the lesions or the skin, alters the computation of the threshold.

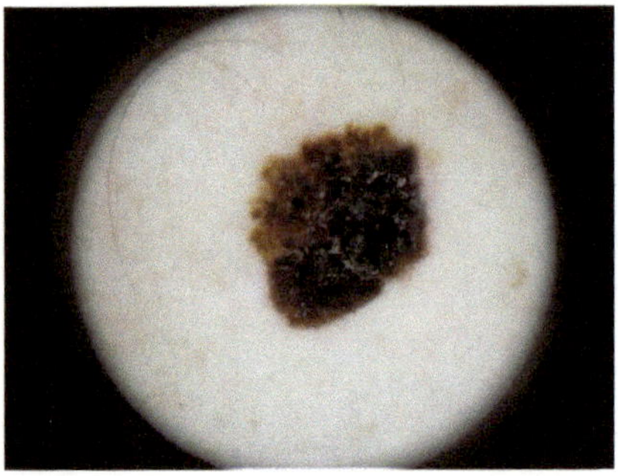

Figure 15. Dermoscopy with the black borders which alters the threshold computation

To solve this problem, and taking into account the characteristics of the location of the lesions, we can apply the Otsu's method to all the image but using only the interior of the image to compute the threshold. This minimizes the influence of the black borders.

Once we have the binarized image, it is advisable to apply *opening* and *closing* morphological operations to relax the borders and eliminate small objects (using *opening* operation) and borders (using *closing* operation). These operations can be applied using *imopen* and *imclose* Matlab functions.

Other Matlab function which can be applied to the binarized image in order to get white objects without black holes is *imfill.* The performance of this function as *imfill(Bw, 'holes')* is shown in figure 16 (before being applied and being applied). In the example, *Bw* refers to the first binarized image shown in figure 16.

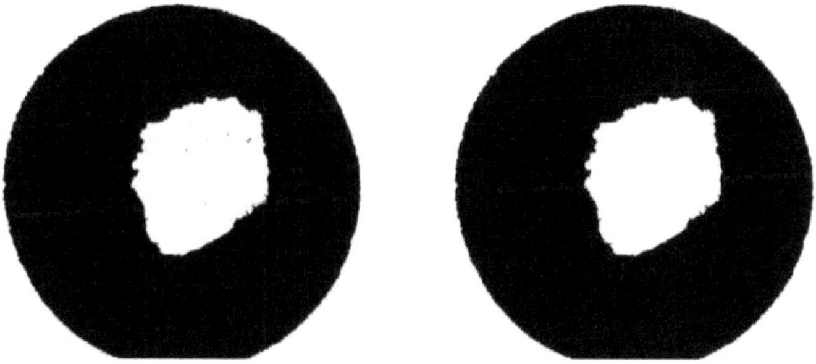

Figure 16. Binarized image before and after *imfill* function is applied

Sometimes this Matlab function generates errors when all the black borders of the original image are connected. This case seems to be a big white object (the borders) with a big hole in the middle (the real dermoscopy). To solve this inconvenience, we can resize the image until we do not obtain only a white object. This is the best wat to ensure the 4 borders are not connected.

Once we have white objects without holes over a black background, the next step is to select the object most centered as the lesion according to the characteristics of the dermoscopies. A very useful Matlab function to do this step is *bwlabel*. This function label all the white objects presented in the image. It returns as many labels as white objects there are in the image.

Now we have to compute the centroids of all the white objects. Since we know which pixels belongs to each object (we know the labels of each pixel) we can apply the equation 3 and then calculate the Euclidean distance from the centroid to the middle of the image according to equation 4.

$$C_x = \frac{\sum_{i=1}^{L} x_i}{L}, C_y = \frac{\sum_{i=1}^{L} y_i}{L} \tag{3}$$

where *Cx* and *Cy* are the coordinates of the centroid, L is the number of pixels which belong to the same object and x*i* and y*i* are the coordinates of each pixel.

$$d_E(P,Q) = \sqrt{(M_x - C_x)^2 + (M_y - C_y)^2} \tag{4}$$

Note that equation 4 is the Euclidean distance for a 2 dimensional space, where M_x and M_y are the coordinates of the middle of the image and C_x and C_y are the coordinates of the computed centroid.

After calculating all the Euclidean distances of each white object from the middle of the image, we can select the label nearest as the lesion. All the pixels with different labels are deleted from the image in order to get a new image with the region of interest in white.

In figure 17 we can observe the result of applying these steps to the image shown in figure 13.

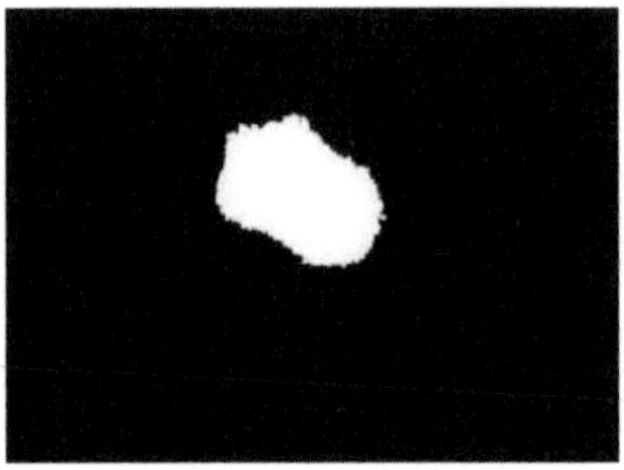

Figure 17. Main object selected after calculating centroids and Euclidean distances

To have a better runtime, is advisable to resize the image around the main object so the feature extraction step is applied to the region of interest and not to the rest of the image. Remember we are working with heavy images.

In figure 18 an example of resizing the image of figure 17 is shown.

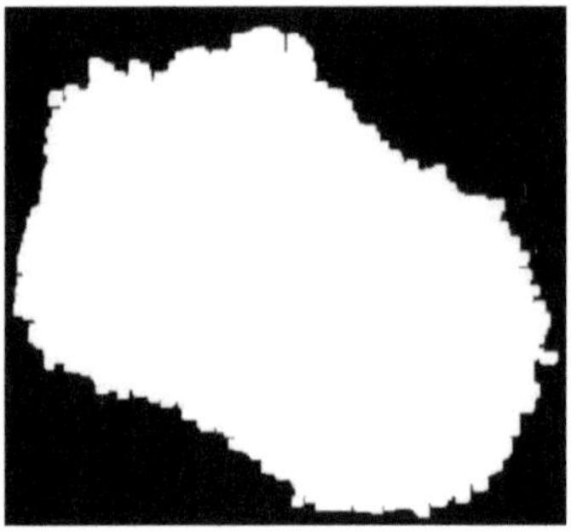

Figure 18. Image obtained after resizing the image of figure 17

3.4.3. Contour extraction

Next step is to obtain the contour of the white object we have selected as region of interest. There are different ways to do this. However, dilation and subtraction could be one of the most intuitive alternatives and gives excellent results.

To dilate the image it is advisable to use a small structural element to not distort the shape of the lesion. In this case we have used *disk* as structural element and we have implemented two consecutives dilations.

Once we have dilated the area of interest, we subtract the original image to the new one, obtaining only the dilated part. We can assume this part as the contour of the lesion.

In figure 19 an example of contour extraction is shown.

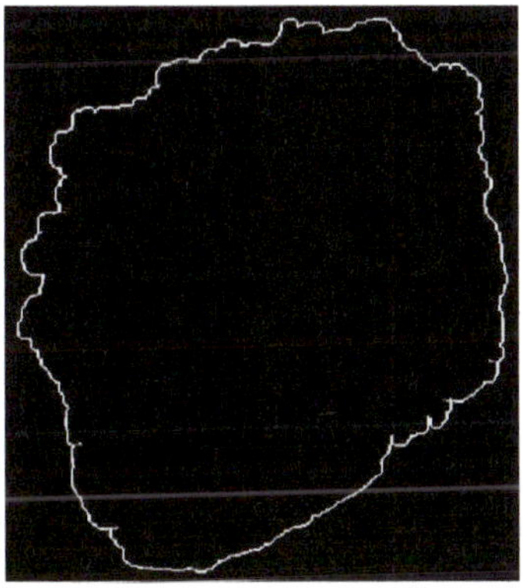

Figure 19. Example of extracted contour

To show the efficacy of this way to get the contour, in figure 20 the contours obtained with two different alternatives of the same algorithm are superposed to the original image.

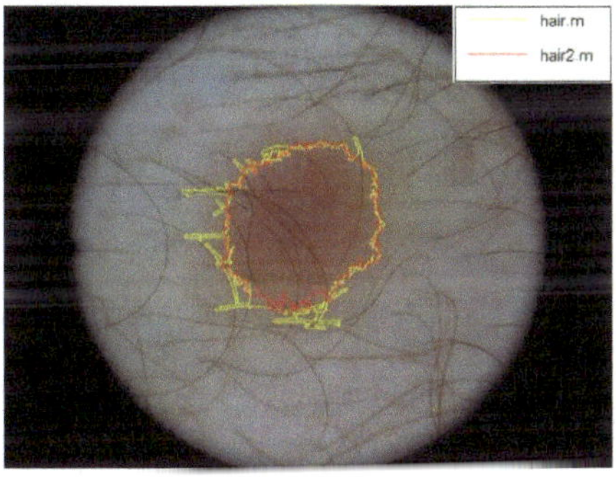

Figure 20. Extracted contours applying different structural elements

4. Feature extraction

In this chapter feature extraction is explained. Later, different feature extraction algorithms are detailed to obtain information about the ACBD rule according to the feature extraction techniques observed in the background.

4.1. Introduction to the feature extraction

A pattern is an entity represented by a vector of features. For example, a pattern can be a sound signal and its vector of features can be the spectral coefficients extracted from it. Another example can be a human face image and numeric characteristics extracted from it.

The best representation of a pattern makes easier taking decision. However, it needs a good knowledge of the problem, what is not always easy.

Feature extraction term has a double meaning. On the one hand it means to extract numeric measures from the data of the pattern. On the other hand, it is also defined as the process to build a group of characteristics (n dimensional) from the input data (m dimensional with m>n).

In general, the objective is the minimum group of characteristics necessary to determine the class of all possible objects. The selected characteristics should have the following 5 properties:

Economy: the algorithm to calculate the characteristics should have a reasonable cost

Velocity: the computing time should not be more than the viability threshold

Independency: characteristics should not be correlated. Correlated characteristics do not give more discriminative information. Covariance can be used to calculate the independency between the characteristics

Reliability: it implies that feature vector of objects of the same class have to give similar values. It is possible when the vector of the same class have a small dispersion.

Discriminant capacity: it can be defined as the need that vectors of objects from different classes have to give different values. This capacity can be measured using Fisher discriminant. This measure uses the averages and the typical deviations of both classes, according to equation 5.

$$F_{ij} = \frac{(m_i - m_j)^2}{\sigma_i^2 + \sigma_j^2} \quad (5)$$

where m_i and m_j are the averages and σ_i and σ_j are the typical deviations of the two classes.

4.2. Feature extraction

In this section we show different features related to ABCD rule which can be obtained for the lesions and some other features.

Remember that we want to develop an automatic classification system based on the rule, but we are not going to apply the formula of the rule. This means we should obtain as many features as necessary to define the patterns, as explained before. The relation with ABCD rule lies on the fact that the features we are extracting are based on its 4 aspects.

Since there is no a perfect solution for the classification problem, readers are encouraged to develop algorithms to obtain different features which could be or not related to ABCD rule.

Once we obtain different features, we have to apply feature selection and then generate the feature vectors to elaborate the patterns and be able to classify the input images.

4.2.1. Asymmetry features

As mentioned in previous chapters, the first evaluation in the ABCD rule is Asymmetry. Below are shown different features which can be extracted from the images to evaluate the asymmetry of the lesion.

Asymmetry feature 1

This feature is the application of the definition of asymmetry for the rule. It means the lesion has to be divided in different axes as shown in the section 2.2.1. Figure 21 shows the possible axis evaluated here.

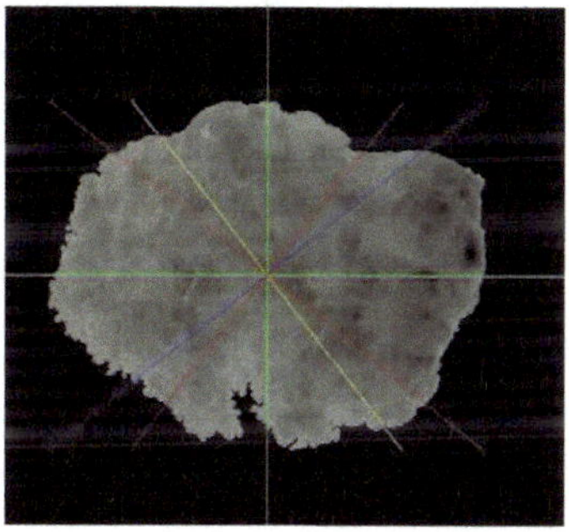

Figure 21. Axis to divide the lesion in order to evaluate its asymmetry

As shown in figure 21, we work with the grayscale image. To have the region out of the lesion in black, we can get the position of black pixels in the image shown in figure 17 and put its values to 0 in the grayscale image. Note that both images have the same size, so the position of the pixels remains equal.

In order to develop the algorithm, the first step is to rotate the image to try to orientate the main body in vertical or horizontal position. This is advisable to make easier the division of the lesion.

Next we can obtain the rectangle with closes the lesion. One way to do this is to obtain the rows and columns of white pixels and select the maximum and minimum of both rows and columns. This gives us the coordinates of the beginning and ending of the region of interest both in vertical and horizontal direction.

Once we have the coordinates of the rectangle, it is easy to obtain the different pairs of axes shown in section 2.2.1. Remember that the pairs are composed of a main axis and its perpendicular.

When we have calculated the different pairs of axes, we have to divide the image to evaluate its asymmetry. This is quiet easy once we have the coordinates of the axes. In figure 22 we can observe the two halves obtained when dividing the image according to its main diagonal.

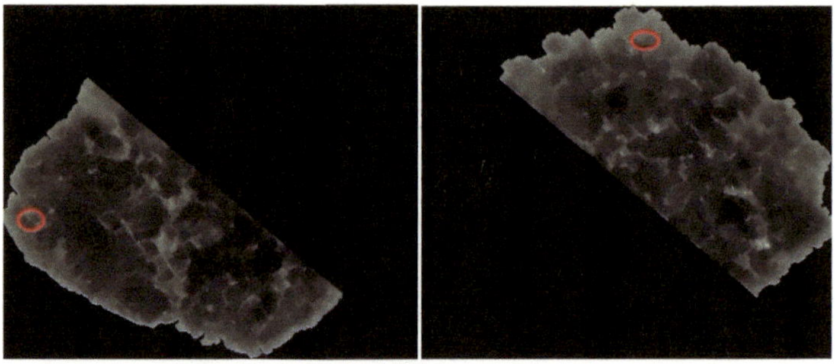

Figure 22. The two halves of a lesion when dividing it by its main diagonal

In red we have highlighted two areas which should be equal if the lesion is symmetric.

Once we have the two halves, we evaluate the asymmetry. It is evaluated according to the color and the area of the lesion. This is possible by evaluating the histograms of both images and computing their areas.

Related to the histograms, we can assume that the black pixels belong to the background since color information is on the gray levels. So we can put to 0 the number of pixels with a value of 0 in the histograms.

For the area, we use the binarized image and compute the number of pixels equal to 1, since we know the lesion is the white object because we have deleted all the rest of possible objects as shown before.

Once we have obtained the areas and histograms similarities of both halves of each image, we label as 0 or 1 both similarities and add the result to the result of the similarities of the other half. For each pair we can obtain a result from 0 to 1. Finally we use as feature the minor score of the three pairs.

The problem appears when deciding to label as 0 or 1 the similarities. We have to set thresholds for both the area and color similarities. This kind of features usually gives problems since we are making decisions according to our visual interpretation about a lesion is or not symmetric.

Asymmetry feature 2

The second proposed feature is the correlation coefficient between the two halves. The main goal of this feature is to obtain information of the distribution of both the color and the area of the lesion.

The initial processing is the same of the previous feature to obtain the different possible pairs. Then, both halves are rotated in order to have the division in the horizontal direction, as shown in figure 23.

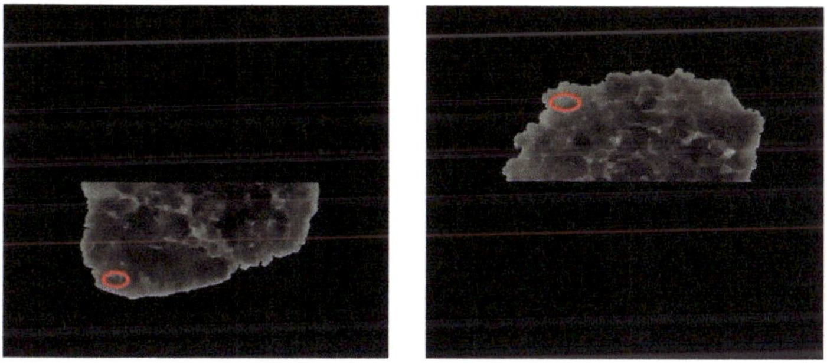

Figure 23. The two halves of a lesion when dividing it by its main diagonal and rotate them

Before applying the correleation, one of the halves has to be inverted to have both halves overlaped. For example, the red areas of the images have to be overlaped once one of them is inverted.

Figure 24 shows the two halves after inverting one of the halves.

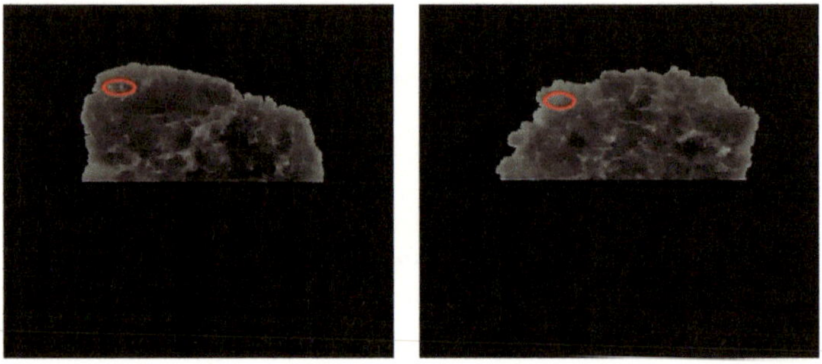

Figure 24. The two halves of a lesion after rotating them and inverting one of the halves

Then we have to obtain the vectors of both images and apply *corrcoef* Matlab function to them.

The result is a value from 0 to 1. 1 is obtained when both vectors are exactly the same. The more different vectors are, the more the result tends to 0. If both vectors have nothing in common, the result is NaN (Not a Number).

According to the different possible pairs, the proposed ones to be used are the horizontal, vertical, main diagonal and secondary diagonal. As features to characterize the lesions, the four coefficients calculated for each of the four possible pairs are used.

4.2.1.1. Border features

This section presents some proposed features to be obtained according to the borders information.

Border feature 1

The first feature is the one related directly with the ABC rule. If we remember the rule, it evaluates the abruptness of the borders. As it was shown, in most of cases the lesion is divided in 8 segments, so the total border score goes from 0 to 8.

One simply way to evaluate the abruptness is modify the threshold applied when binarizing the lesion. If we reduce the threshold, pixels with tonalities near to the older threshold are binarized to white. If these near tonalities are in the borders of the lesion, the area obtained after all the process will be bigger.

In figure 25 we can observe a binarized lesion with the threshold obtained when applying Otsu's method and the one obtained when reducing the threshold the 15%.

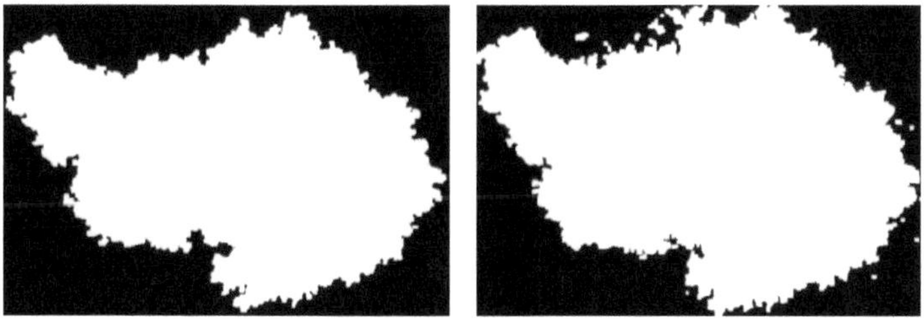

Figure 25. Binarized images when applying Otsu's threshold and the threshold reduced by the 15%

As we can observed, when the threshold has been modified (right picture in figure 25) the area is higher.

Then, if we subtract both images, we obtain the growth of the area due to the reduction of the threshold. We obtain the pixels with a tonality very near to the lesion, so we can conclude they mean there are not abruptness terminations.

Before computing the score, we have to eliminate the isolated objects which not belong to the lesion.

Once we have eliminated them, we have to orientate the lesion, as we did when evaluating the asymmetry and divide the lesion in 8 segments. To divide the lesion, we can use the coordinates we obtained for the horizontal, vertical, main diagonal and secondary diagonal and their perpendicular lines.

In figure 26 we can observe the image once it has been divided in 8 segments.

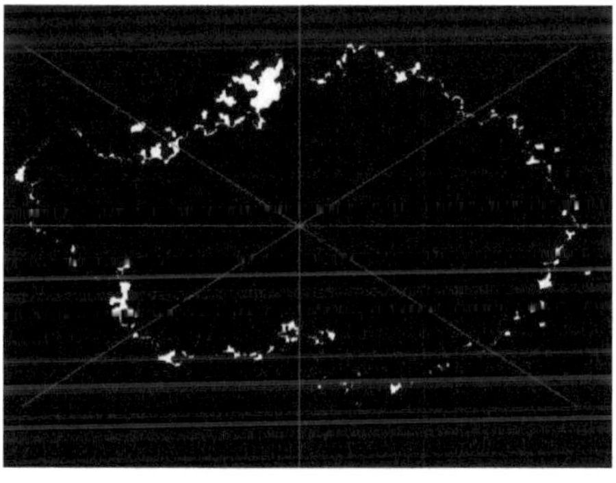

Figure 26. Image after subtracting both binarized images and being divided in 8 segments

Next we have to compute the number of pixels the lesions has grown in each segment. This computation should be related to the number of pixels the original lesion had in the segment we are computing. So we have to obtain 8 percentages which give us the growth in each of the 8 segments.

Finally we have to set a threshold to decide if each of the percentage obtained is high enough to say that the finalization of the border is not abruptness.

The final score of this feature is the sum of the 8 decisions.

Border feature 2

The second feature is based on the sentence "To draw the border of a benign lesion is not necessary to be as Picasso". This sentence means that with a simple stroke we should be able to draw the shape of a benign lesion.

This sentence was said by Dr. Gregorio Carretero in one of the meetings with the doctors at *Hospital Universitario de Gran Canaria Doctor Negrín.*

In other words, the changes of the radius along the lesion should be soft. The ideal mole is totally circular, so its radius does not change along the border of the lesion.

So, this way of extracting border information is based on the computation of the evolution of the radius along the lesion [19]. To do this, we use the image which shows the contour of the lesion, as the one shown in figure 19.

First of all we orientate the original in the horizontal direction. Then we can apply morphological operators as the ones shown previously to try to get a one pixel width contour.

Next, in order to have the coordinates of the border we can use the next code, which gives the coordinates of the external pixels of the contour [22].

```
B = bwboundaries(image, 'no_holes');
for k = 1:length(B)
        boundary = B{k};
end
```

Taking into account the high size of the images we are using, the obtained vector (B) should have a big amount of elements. If we evaluate the changes between surrounding coordinates we are not getting useful information since they are going to be very similar. One possible solution is sampling the vector with a factor of 10. Then we can obtain a general description of the radius evolution.

The next step is to obtain the center of the lesion in order to calculate the radius. To do this we can use the rectangle which contains the lesion. Remember we have already obtained the first and last rows and columns. With this data we can obtain the center of the lesion.

Once we have the coordinates of the points to evaluate and the center of the lesion, we compute the radius by applying the Euclidean distance as shown in equation 4 in section 3.4.2.

If we plot the vector once we have obtained all the distances, we can obtain a graphic as the one shown in figure 27, where *x* axis shows the number of samples evaluated and the *y* axis the radius normalized by the maximum.

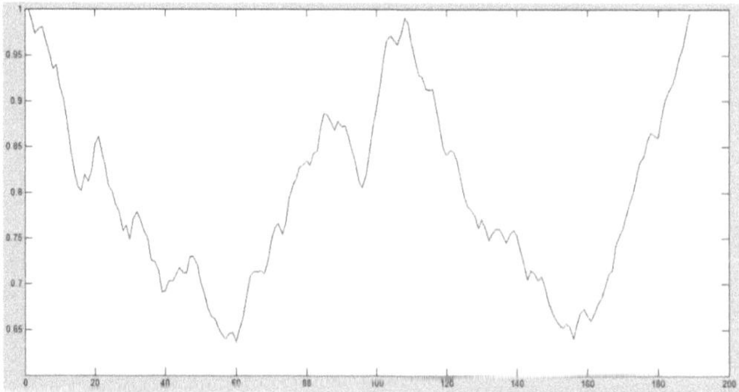

Figure 27. Evolution of the radius along the lesion

One way to characterize the graphic of the figure 27 is to obtain its gradient. We can compute it by using the function *diff* of Matlab. This function returns the differences between a value and the next one.

If we show the obtained vector of differences, we can have a graphic as the one shown in figure 28, where the *x* axis is the number of samples and the *y* axis the difference between the values.

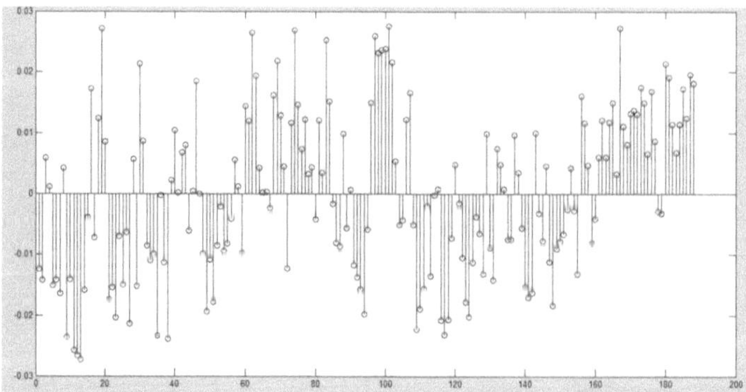

Figure 28. Difference diagram of the radius evolution

In order to obtain the features about the information of the borders, the mean and the standard deviation of this last vector is computed. Notice that the mean and the deviation have to be computed with the absolute values of the vector in order to avoid the possibility of obtaining zero features due to the positive and negative values when the radius is not constant.

For each image we obtain 2 new features which give information about the shape of the lesion.

When evaluating different results obtained for both malign and benign lesions, the radius evolution diagrams look very similar. However, the difference diagrams show some contrasts. The difference diagrams of the benign lesions usually have a lower maximum value than the diagrams of the malign lesions.

4.2.2. Color features

In this section, several features related to the color are presented. These features are extracted in order to obtain information about the third parameter of the ABCD rule (Color). The main difference between the following features is based on the color space used to extract them.

Color feature 1

The first feature is the evaluation of the presence of different colors in the lesion, as evaluated when applying the ABCD rule. So, we have to develop an algorithm to evaluate the presence of different color components in the RGB color space.

The colors to evaluate are dark brown, light brown, black, blue-gray, red and white. The main idea is to define six color regions and label each pixel of the lesion with the label of one of the six groups.

In figure 29 we can observe a lesion before detecting the colors. In figure 30 we can observe the detected colors, which are blue, light and dark brown and black, shown in sub-figures.

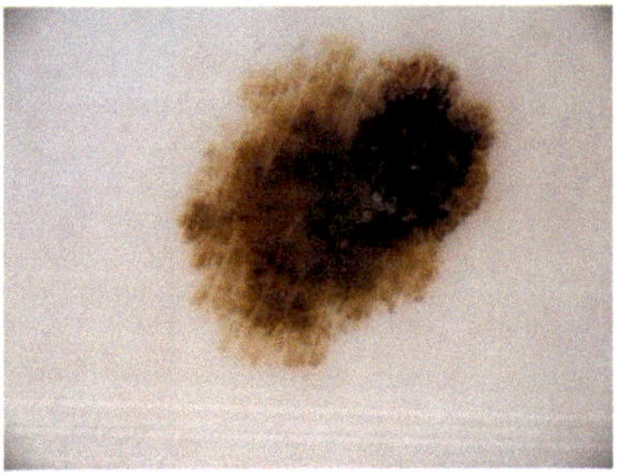

Figure 29. Image to process in order to detect the colors

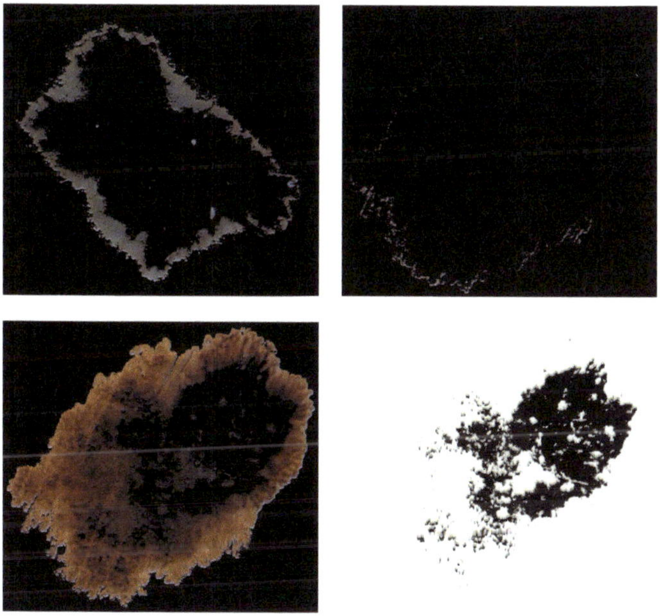

Figure 30. Colors detected in the lesion of the figure 30

When defining the six regions there are some problems. One of them is to set the limit between them, for example, defining when a tonality is light brown and when it is dark brown. We have to set the limits of the six regions according to our perceptions.

Note that when defining the color regions, the user has to set 3 values. Remember RGB space is defined as a 3 dimensional cube, so it has 3 coordinates (R, G and B).

The definition of the regions is a good exercise for the readers in order to notice the difficulty when defining threshold in this kind of automatic classification systems. Note that the final classification depends on the threshold defined. The ideal features should not depend on thresholds defined for the developer, unless the feature is well known and the thresholds are very well-defined by experts.

Color feature 2

This second feature evaluates the histograms of the RGB picture. Remember that a RGB image is formed of 3 sub-pictures, as shown in figure 8. Moreover, each of these 3 sub-pictures is an image represented by a 2 dimensional matrix.

The algorithm to develop should characterize the histograms of the 3 sub-images and the histogram of the grayscale image obtained from the original image.

In figure 31, we can observe the histograms obtained when evaluating the Red channel and the grayscale image of a mole and a melanoma. To obtain the histograms, it is possible to use the function *imhist* of Matlab.

However, the function *imhist* uses both the area of the lesion and the area around the lesion. One way to minimize this error is to use the image with all the pixels which do not belong to the lesion changed to white. Once the histograms have been obtained, the contribution of the white color has to be deleted.

The features are the evaluation of the width of the main lobes of both red, green, blue and red image histograms. The width is computed according to the following formula:

$$\xi = \max(Histogram) - 2 * \sigma(Histogram) \tag{6}$$

where ξ is the result, max(Histogram) is the highest value of the Histogram (in this case it is 1 since it is normalized) and σ is the standard deviation. ξ-formula has been obtained as a solution to characterize the histogram by following a heuristic method [1].

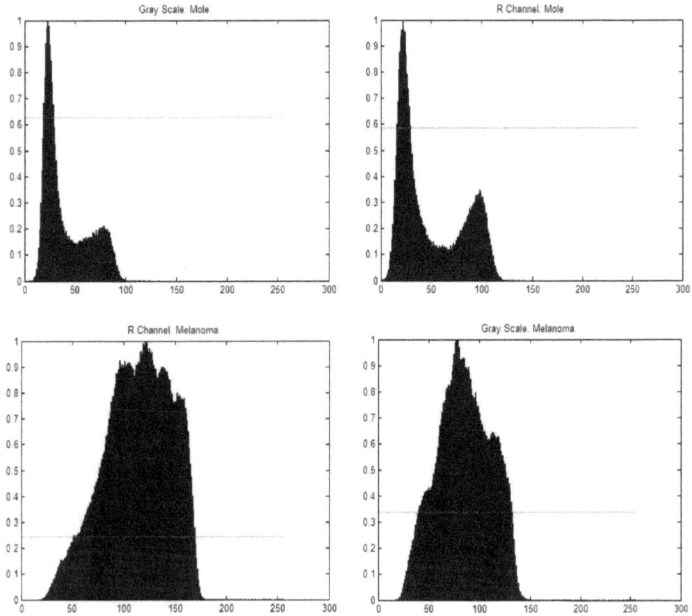

Figure 31. Histograms of the Red channel and grayscale image of a mole (1st row) and a melanoma (2nd row)

Color feature 3

This feature is also based on the RGB color space. In this case, R, G and B components are separated into 3 different vectors. Each of these vectors is evaluated by calculating its maximum and minimum values, means and standard deviations.

Color feature 4

Using again RGB color space, it is possible to obtain the relative chromaticity of the image. According to [15], this feature reduces the light variation and equalizes the individuals variations of each subject.

This feature is computed for each of the three RGB components according to the following formula:

$$CR_i = \frac{\mu^i_{RGB}}{\sum_{i=\{R,G,B\}} \mu^i_{RGB}} - \frac{\nu^i_{RGB}}{\sum_{i=\{R,G,B\}} \nu^i_{RGB}} \qquad (7)$$

where μ is the mean of the RGB channels inside the area of the lesion and ν is the mean of RGB channels in the area around the lesion.

Color feature 5

In this occasion, we should repeat the algorithm develop for the color feature 3, using the HSI (Hue, Saturation, Intensity) color space instead of the RGB color space. In figure 32 we can observe a lesion represented using the HIS color space.

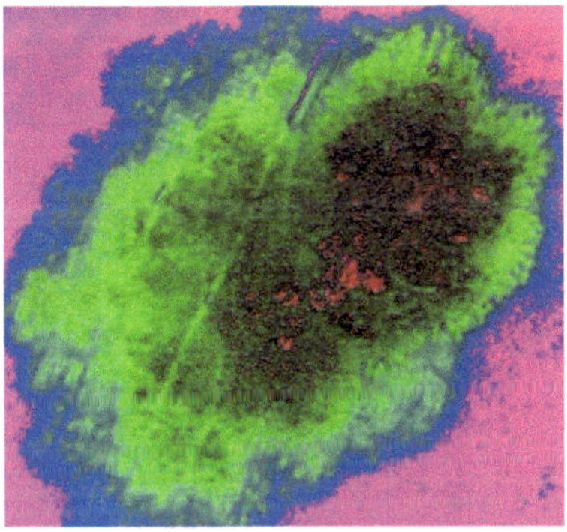

Figure 32. Lesion represented using the HSI color space

To obtain the HSI color space, the algorithm shown below can be applied to the RGB color space image according to the examples available in Mathworks website.

```
num = 0.5*((R-G)+(R-B));
den = sqrt((R-G).^2+(R-B).*(G-B));
angle = acos(num./(den+eps));
H = angle;
H(B>G) = 2*pi-H(B>G);
H = H/(2*pi);
num = min(min(R,G),B);
den = R+G+B;
den(den==0) = eps;
S = 1-3.*num./den;
H(S==0) = eps;
I = (R+G+B)/3;
HSI_Image = cat(3,H,S,I)
```

In the HSI case, S channel is not evaluated since it gives no information. Moreover, H and I channels have to be normalized because they depend on the tone of the skin around the lesion. For H and I normalized channels, maximum and minimum values, median and standard values are obtained.

Color feature 6

For this sixth color feature, HSV (Hue, Saturation, Value) color space is used in order to obtain the maximum, minimum, mean and standard deviation values, as explained in color features 3 and 5.

To obtain the HSV image from the RGB image, we can use the Matlab function *rgb2hsv*, which applies transformations to the RGB channels, as shown in the case of the HSI color space. To know the applied transformations, take a look to the information of the named function.

In figure 33 we can observe a lesion represented in the HSV color space.

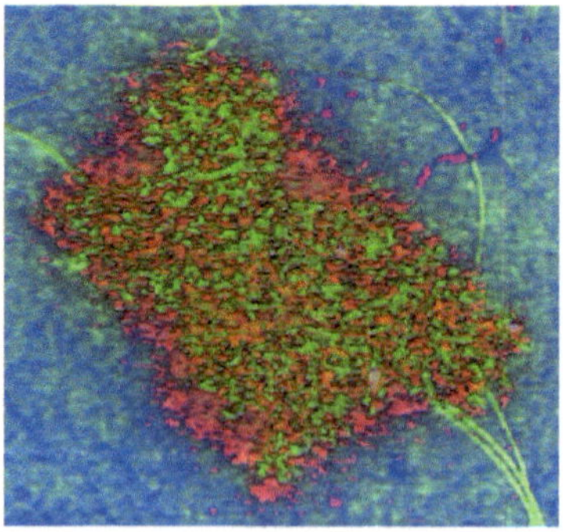

Figure 33. Lesion represented using the HSV color space

In this case, the mean value of each of the three color components gives no practical information, so it is not used as feature of the lesion.

Color feature 7

In this case, the same characterization used in the previous color feature is applied to the L*A*b color space. To obtain the representation of the image in this new color space, the following transformation can be applied to the RGB components [17].

L = sqrt(R.^2+G.^2+B.^2)
A = acos(B/L)
b = acos(R/(L*sin(A)))

In figure 34, a lesion represented using the Lab space color is shown.

Figure 34. Lesion represented using the LAb color space

4.2.3. Texture features

As fourth group of features to characterize the lesions, we can use the texture of the lesion. Remember the difficulty of evaluating the presence of dermatoscopic structures in the lesion, according to the ABCD rule, and the alternative of evaluating the texture to obtain information about it[16].

The evaluation of the texture can be done by the computation of the histograms of the magnitude and the phase of the gradient of the lesion. To obtain the gradient, we can apply the following procedure [1,16]:

1. From RGB channels, we select the one with the highest entropy, i.e., the most informative channel. The entropy is measured according to the next equation [27].

$$H = -\sum_{i} p_i(k) * \log_2 p_i(k) \qquad (8)$$

where $p_i(k)$ denotes the probability of the i−th color channel being equal to k at a lesion pixel x. This distribution can be easily obtained by computing the histogram of each color channel inside the lesion.

2. The gray level image of the selected channel is filtered using a Gaussian filter with $\sigma=2$, and then the gradient vector is computed at each point $g(x) = [g_1(x)\ g_2(x)]^T$ using Sobel masks.

3. The gradient magnitude and orientation are then computed as usual:

$$\| g(x) \| = \sqrt{g_1^2(x) + g_2^2(x)} \tag{9}$$

$$\theta(x) = \tan^{-1}\left(\frac{g_2(x)}{g_1(x)} \right) \tag{10}$$

Operator g(x) is used with two 3×3 kernels which are convolved with the original image to calculate approximations of the derivatives - one for horizontal changes $g_1(x)$, and one for vertical $g_2(x)$.

The gradient magnitude and orientation are then characterized by their histograms, using $M_a=10$ and $M_\theta=40$ bins, respectively.

As examples, gradient magnitude obtained for a melanoma and a mole are shown in figure 35, respectively.

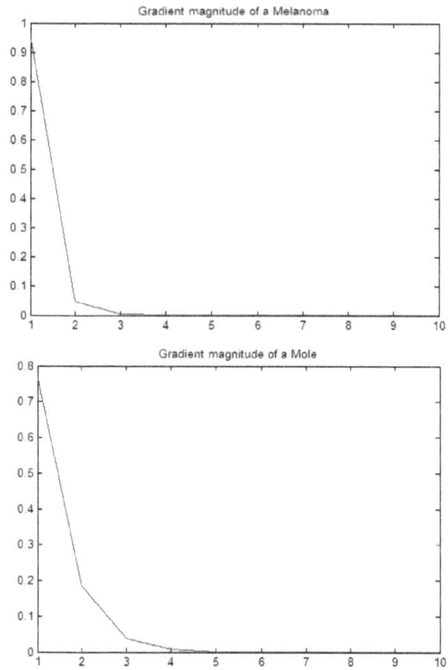

Figure 35. Gradient magnitude for a melanoma and for a mole

4.2.4. Other features

Independently of the ABCD rule parameters, in this section we shown some used geometrical features which can be extracted from the lesions in order to obtain more information [28].

Circularity index (CRC): It explains the shape uniformity

$$CRC = \frac{4*A*\pi}{P^2} \tag{11}$$

Irregularity index (Ir):

$$Ir = \frac{P}{A} \tag{12}$$

where P is the perimeter and A the area of the lesion.

5. Classifier

Once the features have been obtained, the reader has to choose what classifier use. There are several well-known classifiers as Support Vector Machines, Neural Networks, etc. The selection should be based on the characteristics of the problem the user wants to solve.

In this case, we have used Support Vector Machines. Some known bibliography to get the knowledge to use this classifier is available in [29-31].

Reading the available bibliography is enough to get the basis to manage with this classifier and modify the designing parameters to run different simulations in order to obtain good results.

Because of this reason, we focus this chapter in other points the user can modify to adapt the classifier to the problem. In the next chapter we will show the modifications we have implemented in our solution.

First of all, due to the small size of the database, we decided to apply leave-one out validation method. It was repeated for all the 48 samples. Leave-one out validation was applied according to [32].

As it is known, in the test, once the samples are compared with the models obtained for each of the training classes, we obtain similarities between the testing samples and the models.

One of the possibilities of modification consists on the way of labeling the testing samples according to the models. The normal classification consists in labeling the testing sample according to the highest similarity.

6. Feature selection

The main idea of feature selection is to obtain the features which give discriminant information; it is mean they give information to be able to distinguish between the classes.

As we have obtained a lot of different features, many of them possibly give no discriminant information. One way to visually measure the information is to use *boxplot* diagrams.

These diagrams represent the distribution of a feature for the studied classes. In this case we obtain diagrams with two boxes, one per each of the two classes. The main boxes of the diagrams represent the median and the first and third quartiles of the distribution, as shown in figure 36.

In figure 37 we observe an example of a boxplot diagram obtained for two classes.

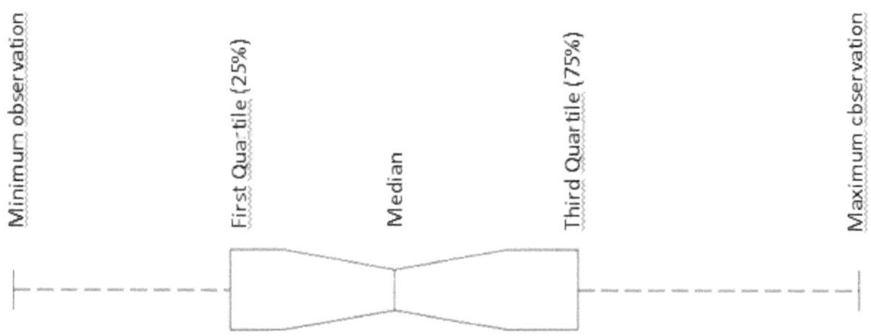

Figure 36. Example of boxplot diagram

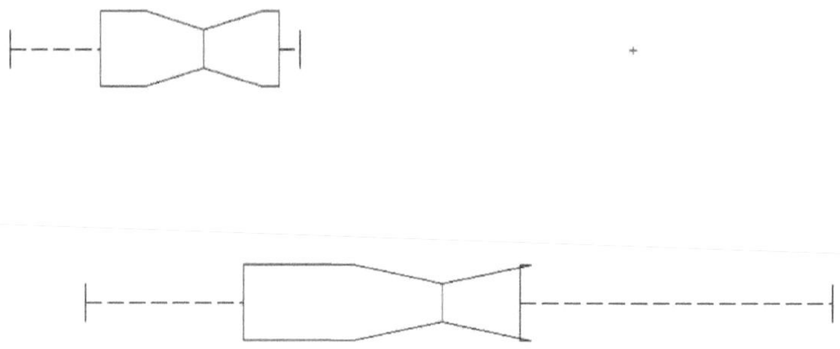

Figure 37. Example of boxplot diagram for two classes

The ideal feature should give a diagram where the boxes are not overlapped. This would mean the feature gives discriminant information.

We encourage the readers to obtain the boxplot diagrams for the extracted features in order to evaluate their information. In our case we obtain always overlapped diagrams, so there is any feature able to discriminate independently to the others.

Another possibility is to study the combination of two features. To do this we can represent each lesion in a bidimensional space where the axis are the values obtained for the two studied features. In this case we can obtain plots as the one shown in figure 38.

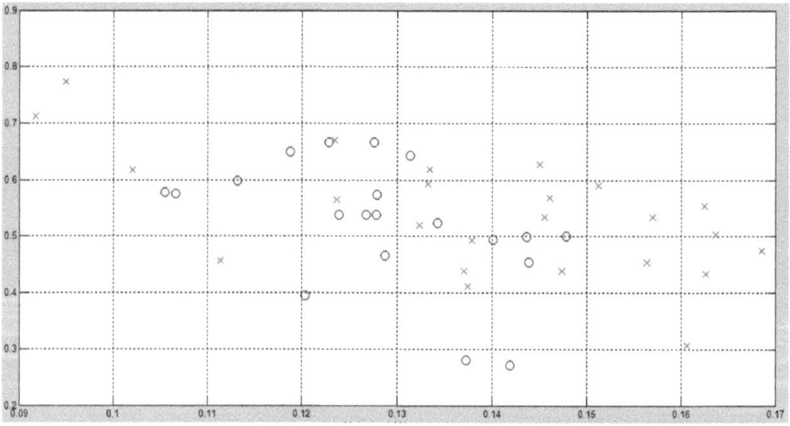

Figure 38. Plot obtained when representing each lesion with two features

In this case, the ideal plot should show two separated regions, one for each of the two classes. In the studies cases we have not obtained this ideal representation.

It is also possible to study a combination of three features by visual inspection. In this case we would obtain representations for the lesions in a three dimensional space. Again, the ideal case should show two different areas. We do not show any example since it is difficult to observe the three dimensional space in a picture.

Apart from the visual inspection, a classifier can be used to apply feature selection. The user can run a simulation with all the features, independently of the others and select the feature which gives the best result. Next, run simulation with this feature and a second features, as many times as possible second features the user has, and select the best pair of features. Next create group of three features using the best pair of features.

The simulation can stop when no improvement is gotten.

There a lot of bibliography about the feature extraction. There is no supposed to be a better technique, however applying all the possible techniques is a tedious task.

In this case we have obtained two groups of features which give good partial results by applying random group creation.

In table number 5 we can observe a brief description and the number of features which form the 2 feature sets.

Feature set	Description of the features	Number of features
1	Color evaluations using RGB, HSV, HSI and CIE Lab color spaces Evaluation of module and phase of image's gradient	36
2	Radius evolution along the lesion Geometric features	6

Table 5. Characteristics of the feature sets

7. Results

In this chapter we show the results obtained for the two feature sets mentioned in the previous chapter. Next we will show a modification applied to the labelling method which give better results.

Finally we propose a classification tree system as system to get a high sensitivity together to the alternative labeling method. A sensitivity of 100% means that all the patients with melanoma are identified.

7.1. Sensitivity and specificity

The results are evaluated based on the values of accuracy, sensitivity and specificity. These values are obtained according to the following equations [33]:

$$Accuracy = \frac{TruePositives + TrueNegatives}{TruePositives + TrueNegatives + FalsePositives + FalseNegatives} \tag{13}$$

$$Sensitivity = \frac{TruePositives}{TruePositives + FalseNegatives} \tag{14}$$

$$Specificity = \frac{TrueNegatives}{TrueNegatives + FalsePositives} \tag{15}$$

Our point of view tries to emphasize the medical aspect of automatic cancer diagnosis, where false negatives are not allowed. This means a high sensitivity is desired.

7.2. Alternative labelling method

SVM assigns a label to the testing sample according to the similarity between the sample and the Support Vectors generated for each of the two classes.

As we have mentioned before, one way to modify the Support Vector Machine classifier is the labelling method. It is means, do not label the samples depending on the highest similarity.

In this particular case, we work with two classes. This means only two labels are possible (+1 and -1) as this is a bi-class algorithm

However, an alternative labeling method can be applied. The proposed method looks for a higher sensitivity by labeling the samples as malign lesions when the difference between the obtained similarities is lower than a given threshold. It other words, samples are labeled as malign when there is doubt about its nature.

One option to evaluate the optimal threshold is calculating ROC curves, as the one shown in figure 39. This curve is useful to evaluate the point where the false acceptances and the false rejections are equals. This point is supposed to be used as the threshold.

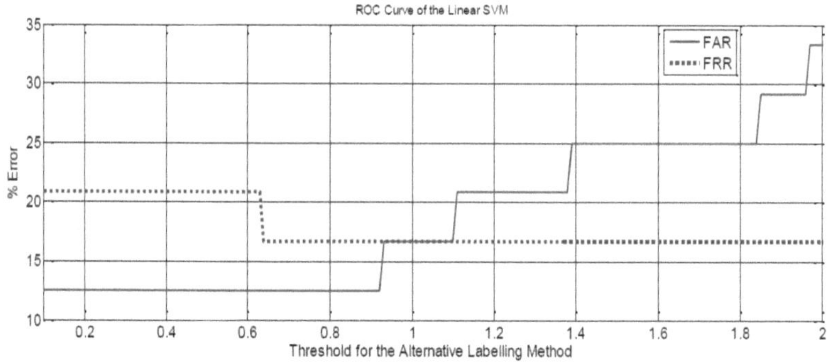

Figure 39. ROC curve of the Linear Support Vector Machine

7.3. Partial results

As there is no interest in the particulars results obtained for the two sets evaluated since it depends on the classifier and the features used, in table 6 we show the results obtained for the second set when using difference thresholds for the alternative labelling method for the same type of classifier.

Classifier	Threshold	Sensitivity	Specificity	Accuracy	Gamma
Gaussian kernel	0.15	91.66%	66.66%	79.16%	4×10^{-6}
Gaussian kernel	0.10	91.66%	70.83%	81.25%	4×10^{-6}
Gaussian kernel	0.01	87.50%	75.00%	81.25%	4×10^{-6}

Table 6. Results when Gaussian kernel is used with feature set number 2

Gamma is the value of the inverse of the Gaussian kernel's standard deviation which gives better results in our case.

Another remarkable point is the fact that both feature set give good results for different types of Support Vector Machine. In table 7 we can observe the best performance for both sets.

Classifier	Threshold	Sensitivity	Specificity	Accuracy	Gamma
Linear	1.00	83.33%	83.33%	83.33%	---
Gaussian kernel	0.10	91.66%	70.83%	81.25%	4×10^{-6}

Table 7. Chosen configurations for each of the classifiers

As shown in table 7, the first feature set uses a Linear Support Vector Machine while the second one uses a Support Vector Machine with a Gaussian kernel.

If we choose one classifier and its feature set we would have not very good results since the sensitivity is less than 92% and the accuracy is always under 84%. However, in our case, studying the lesions which are bad labeled, we observe that both classifiers fails when labelling different lesions.

This fact is the base of the system proposed in the next section.

7.4. Classification tree system

A decision tree is a good option to implement a system robust for noisy data [34]. If we choose one classifier and its feature set we would have not very good results since the sensitivity is less than 92% and the accuracy is always under 84%. However, in our case, studying the lesions which are bad labeled, we observe that both classifiers fails when labelling different lesions.

In this case, the tree consists on applying the two tests to all the testing samples, obtaining two labels for each testing sample, as shown in figure 40.

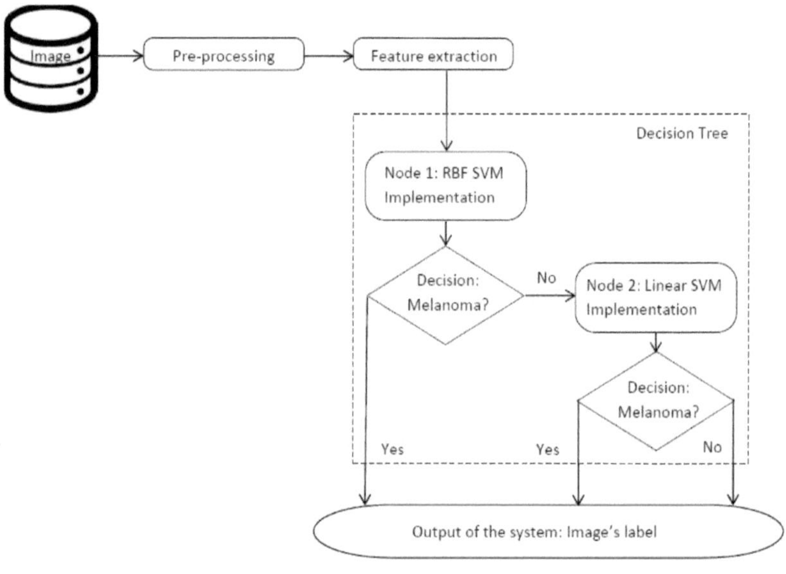

Figure 40. Classification tree system

The final label is the strictest one, so if one of the classifiers labels the sample as melanoma, the final label is melanoma.

An option to optimize runtime is applying the second classifier only when the first one produces a benign label.

This method, together to the alternative labelling method, increases the sensitivity of the system.

7.5. Global results

Once we have shown the alternative labelling method and the results obtained for both classifiers when using it, in table 8 the final performance when we apply the classification tree using both classifiers is shown.

Sensitivity	Specificity	Accuracy
100%	66.66%	83.33%

Table 8. Results of the classification tree system

In table 9 we can observe the True positives, False Positives, True Negatives and False Negatives obtained for both the two classifiers and the tree system.

Classifier	TP	FP	TN	FN
Linear	20	4	20	4
Gaussian kernel	22	7	17	2
Final system	24	8	16	0

Table 9. Results for each of the classifiers and the final system

In conclusion, the classification system has been designed as a decision tree with two different SVM classifiers, one with linear kernel and the other one using RBF kernel. The success rates are around 83.33%. However, the system gets a sensitivity of 100%, what means no false negatives are allowed. This fact is a good point for the system from the point of view of the medical application.

Another interpretation of the results is that using this approach, a second opinion is given and 66.66% of biopsies could be avoided.

References

[1] E. Guerra-Segura, C. Travieso-González, J. Alonso-Hernández, A. Ravelo-García, and G. Carretero, "Symmetry Extraction in High Sensitivity Melanoma Diagnosis," *Symmetry (Basel).*, vol. 7, pp. 1061–1079, 2015.

[2] E. Perera, N. Gnaneswaran, and R. Jennens, "Malignant Melanoma," *Healthcare*, vol. 2, pp. 1–19, 2014.

[3] E. Garraway, H. Widlund, and M. A. Rubin, "Integrative genomic analyses identify MITF as a lineage survival oncogene amplified in malignant melanoma," *Nature*, vol. 436, pp. 117–122, 2005.

[4] B. Garcia, A. Mendez, I. Ruiz, G. Nunez, and A. Abtane, "Skin Cancer Parameterization algorithm based on epiluminiscence image processing," in *IEEE International Symposium on Signal Processing and Information Technology (ISSPIT)*, pp. 236–241.

[5] P. Rutkowski, M. Zdzienicki, Z. I. Nowecki, and A. C. J. van Akkooi, "Surgery of Primary Melanomas," *Cancers (Basel).*, vol. 2, pp. 824–841, 2010.

[6] E. Guerra, C. M. Travieso, J. B. Alonso, and G. Carretero, "An image segmentation technique for melanocytic diseases classification in dermoscopy images," in *I Congreso de Jóvenes Investigadores de Canarias*, 2015, pp. 41–44.

[7] P. Malvehy and S. Puig, *Principios de Dermatoscopia.* Barcelona, Spain, 2002.

[8] N. M. Sirakov, M. Mete, and N. S. Chakrader, "Automatic boundary detection and symmetry calculation in dermoscopy images of skin lesions," in *18th IEEE International Conference on Image Processin (ICIP)*, 2011, pp. 1605–1608.

[9] B. Amaliah, C. Fatichah, and R. Rahmat, "ABCD feature extraction of image dermatoscopic based on morphology analysis for melanoma skin cancer diagnosis," *J. Ilmu Komput. Inf*, vol. 3, pp. 82–90, 2010.

[10] I. Guyon and S. D. Barnhill, "System and Method for Remote Melanoma Screening," WO/2011/087807, 2011.

[11] G. Capdehourart, A. Corez, A. Bazzano, and P. Muse, "Pigmented Skin Lesions Classification Using Dermatoscopic Images," in *Progress in Pattern Recognition, Image Analysis, Computer Vision, and Applications*, vol. 5856, Berlin, Germany: Springer, 2009, pp. 537–544.

[12] K. M. Clawson, P. J. Morrow, B. W. Scotney, D. J. McKenna, and O. M. Dolan, "Determination of optimal axes for skin lesion asymmetry quantification," in *IEEE International Conference on Image Processing*, 2007, pp. 453–456.

[13] T. Tanaka, R. Yamada, M. Tanaka, K. Shimizu, M. Tanaka, and H. Oka, "A Study on the Image Diagnosis of Melanoma," in *26th Annual International Conference of the IEEE Engineering in Medicine and Biology Society*, 2004, pp. 1597–1600.

[14] A. Parolin, E. Herzer, and C. R. Jung, "Semi-Automated Diagnosis of Melanoma through the Analysis of Dermatological Images," in *23rd SIBGRAPI Conference on Graphics, Patterns and Images (SIBGRAPI)*, 2010, pp. 71–78.

[15] B. Kusumoputro and A. Ariyanto, "Neural network diagnosis of malignant skin cancers using principal component analysis as a preprocessor," in *IEEE International Joint Conference on Neural Networks*, 1998, pp. 310–315.

[16] J. S. Marques, C. Barata, and T. Mendonc, "On the Role of Texture and Color in the Classification of Dermoscopy Images," in *34th Annual International Conference of the IEEE EMBS*, 2012, pp. 4402–4405.

[17] M. Maragoudakis and I. Maglogiannis, "Skin Lesion Diagnosis from Images Using Novel Ensemble Classification Techniques," in *10th IEEE International Conference on Information Technology and Applications in Biomedicine (ITAB)*, 2010, pp. 1–5.

[18] A. Baldi, M. Quartulli, R. Murace, E. Dragonetti, M. Manganaro, O. Guerra, and S. Bizzi, "Automated Dermoscopy Image Analysis of Pigmented Skin Lesions," *Cancers (Basel).*, vol. 2, pp. 262–273, 2010.

[19] R. Garnavi, M. Aldeen, and J. Bailey, "Computer-Aided Diagnosis of Melanoma Using Border and Wavelet-Based Texture Analysis," *IEEE Trans. InformationTechnology Biomed.*, vol. 16, pp. 1239–1252, 2012.

[20] N. Nguyena, T. Lee, and M. Atkinsa, "Segmentation of Light and Dark Hair in Dermoscopic Images: A Hybrid Approach Using a Universal Kernel," *Med. Imaging 2010 Image Process.*, vol. 7623, 2010.

[21] E. Zagrouba and W. Barjoumi, "An Accelerated System for Melanoma Diagnosis Based on Subset Feature Selection," *J. Comput. Inf. Technol*, vol. 1, pp. 69–82, 2005.

[22] R. C. Gonzalez, R. E. Woods, and S. L. Eddins, *Digital Image Processing Using MATLAB*. Upper Saddle River, NJ, USA: Pearson Prentice Hall, 2004.

[23] MathWorks, "Image Thresholding and Image Segmentation." [Online]. Available: http://www.mathworks.es. [Accessed: 01-Oct-2013].

[24] M. Sezgin and B. Sankur, "Survey over image thresholding techniques and quantitative performance evaluation," *J. Electron. Imaging*, vol. 13, pp. 146–165, 2004.

[25] J. Semmlow, *Biosignal and Biomedical Image Processing, MATLAB-Based Applications*, Signal Pro. CRC Press, 2004.

[26] N. Otsu, "A threshold selection method from gray level histograms," *IEEE Trans. Syst. Man Cybernet*, vol. 9, pp. 62–66, 1979.

[27] C. E. Shannon, "A Mathematical Theory of Communication," *Bell Syst. Tech. J.*, vol. 27, pp. 379–423, 623–656.

[28] I. Maglogiannis and D. I. Kosmopoulosb, "Computational vision systems for the detection of malignant melanoma," *Oncol. Rep.*, pp. 1027–1032, 2006.

[29] C. Cortes and V. Ñ. Vapnik, "Support vector networks," *Mach. Learn.*, vol. 20, pp. 273–297, 1995.

[30] C. J. C. Burges, "A Tutorial on Support Vector Machines for Pattern Recognition," in *Data Mining and Knowledge Discovery*, Amsterdam, The Netherlands: Kluwer Academic Publishers, 1998, pp. 121–167.

[31] G. A. Betancour, "Las Máquinas de Soporte Vectorial (SVMs)," *Sci. Tech.*, no. 27, pp. 67–72, 2005.

[32] S. Arlot, "A survey of cross-validation procedures for model selection," *Static Surv*, vol. 4, pp. 40–79, 2010.

[33] Z. Wen, Z. Nancy, and W. Ning, "Sensitivity, Specificity, Accuracy, Associated Confidence Interval and ROC Analysis with Practical SAS Implementations," in *NESUG proceedings: health care and life sciences*, 2010, pp. 1–9.

[34] J. I. Olszewska, "Automatic Image Annotation based On Multi-Layered Active Contours and Decision Trees," *Int. J. Adv. Comput. Sci. Appl.*, vol. 4, no. 8, pp. 201–208, 2013.